Healing Nourishment for The Heart

Delicious, heart-friendly recipes that are simple to prepare at home

Emily Simmons

Published by The Heirs Publishing Company, 2018.

HEALING NOURISHMENT FOR THE HEART

First edition. October 26, 2018.

Copyright © 2018 Emily Simmons.

ISBN: 978-1393576129

Written by Emily Simmons.

Alcoholism, Twelve-Step Programs
Healing Nourishment for The Heart; Sustenance for The Soul

Delicious, heart-friendly recipes that are simple to prepare at home

Introduction:

Many foods can help to keep your heart healthy, and can even help to undo some of the damage done by poor lifestyle and habits. Certain foods have been shown to lower your blood pressure or cholesterol. Who wouldn't want that? This book aims to present you with recipes for delicious, easy to prepare meals and snacks, that have been especially modified to be healthier for your heart, and your whole body in general, than their traditional counterparts.

So congratulations on your purchase of a book that I hope will not only bring you much pleasure in the kitchen, but also add many more healthy, active years to your life!

Most of us are busy and have little time for food preparation, so my aim has been to keep the recipes short and simple. Some can be frozen for later use, which is always a bonus.

A few of the top foods known to enhance heart health are highlighted for your information here:

Oily fish are among the best foods for heart-health. **Salmon, tuna, sardines** and **mackerel** are a few examples. You'll find recipes that use some of these fish in this book, helping you to easily incorporate them into your diet. Aim to have them at least twice a week.

Walnuts are known to cut your heart disease risk by 50%, and you need just 140g a week. So use them in your breakfast cereal, in salads, and as a healthy snack. **Almonds** and **cashews** are great too.

Berry fruits such as **raspberries, strawberries**, and **blackberries** are loaded with antioxidants such as vitamin C, and with fibre. They have been linked in studies to fewer heart attacks and strokes. So treat yourself to some delicious desserts and breakfasts made with these.

Low fat milk and **yoghurt** are high in potassium, which lowers blood pressure, and low in saturated fats. On the subject of potassium, **bananas** and **potatoes** are high in this mineral too. Speaking of yoghurt, an interesting study done in Japan showed that yoghurt lowers the risk of gum disease, which can in turn cause a higher risk of heart disease. The probiotics in the yoghurt stop the growth of "bad" bacteria in the mouth.

Chickpeas, as well as **beans** and **lentils**, are a good source of soluble fibre- perfect for lowering "bad" LDL cholesterol, and are a base for many delicious meals and snacks. Try the yummy chickpea spread recipe in this book, instead of making a fat laden dip for your next party. Be sure to rinse them in fresh water if you buy them canned, as too much salt can raise your blood pressure, and the canning liquid contains salt. The same goes for canned lentils and beans. Soluble fibre is also found in eggplants (brinjals), apples, and pears.

Oatmeal and **barley** are well-known for lowering LDL cholesterol in the blood. Barley forms the base for one of the soups in this book, and for a filling summer salad, while oats are used for creamy breakfast porridge and some muffins.

Everyone knows that the Mediterranean diet is one of the healthiest ways in the world to eat, and olive oil is a foundational ingredient in this way of cooking. It's used in several recipes here. Use extra-virgin when the distinctive flavour is desired, and a milder version where it needs to be subtler.

Yay! Who would have known it but **chocolate** is good for your heart! (Not to mention your soul.) However, it must be dark chocolate-the darker the better. It's made from cacao, a plant high in flavanols, which help to lower blood pressure and prevent the formation of blood clots. A bonus: dark chocolate can help LDL cholesterol from attaching itself to the artery walls. So, go on, indulge now and then!

Avocados- creamy and luxurious, they are high in "good" oils, which help to lower LDL cholesterol. Enjoy them in salads, in wraps, or even just mashed onto a slice of whole-wheat toast with a squeeze of lemon juice. Try the easy recipe for guacamole in this book.

Red grapes are an excellent addition to any heart-friendly diet. They contain an antioxidant which prevents blood clots (resveratrol.) It's also found in **red wine** and **dark chocolate**, so both of these are good for you in moderation.

Basically, most studies agree that a diet high in vegetables, fruits, low-fat dairy and wholegrains and low in salt, sugar, and saturated fats is the best way to go to prevent or control heart disease. So load your plate with vegetables and fruit, add some wholegrain starch such as brown rice or whole-wheat pasta, and add a small serving of lean protein such as chicken breast or salmon. What could be easier?

SOUPS

Soups are so useful- they can be made in a big batch and then frozen for another day when you are too busy to cook. They're also great for packing into a thermos flask to take to work, instead of buying greasy takeaways during the day when things get busy. A good tip for getting more heart-helping vegetables into your diet is to make a habit of having a bowl of light, vegetable based soup before your main meal.

Most of the recipes we've given you here are wonderful in that they are "meals in one" so you can make a complete meal of them, and feel full, satisfied and very virtuous at the end of it, because you will have had a scrumptious combination of protein, lots of veg, and a few healthy carbs. Combine your bowl of soup with some fresh crusty whole grain bread, and you have a meal fit for a king!

Tomato, Lentil, and Chickpea Soup

Packed with tangy Mediterranean flavors and ingredients, this soup is sure to be a winner on your winter menu. The ingredients are easy to store in your cupboard, too. Serve with fresh, crusty wholegrain bread.

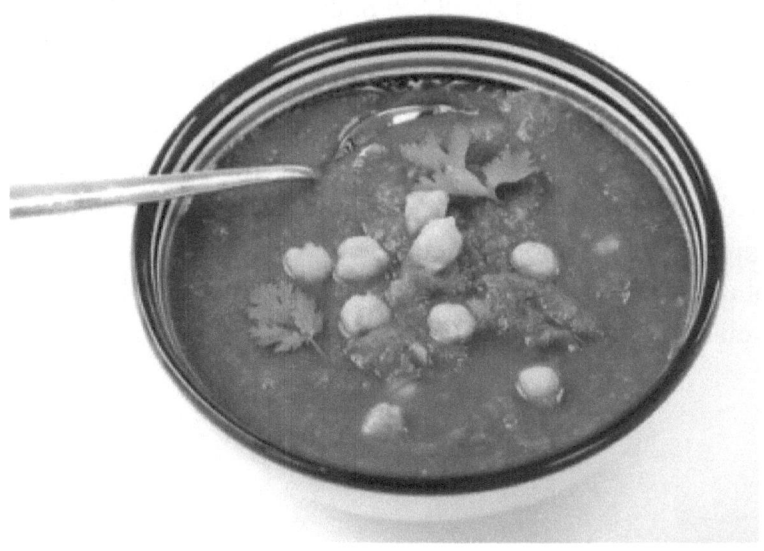

INGREDIENTS:
- 2 tablespoons olive oil
- 1 onion, peeled and finely chopped
- I can kidney beans, drained and rinsed
- 1 can lentils, drained and rinsed
- 1 can chickpeas, drained and rinsed
- 1 can chopped tomatoes
- 1 carrot, peeled and diced
- 2 cloves garlic, finely chopped
- 2 litres unsalted chicken stock
- black pepper to season
- 2 tablespoons fresh Italian parsley, finely chopped

INSTRUCTIONS:

Heat the oil in a large soup pot and lightly brown the onion, carrot, and garlic before adding the beans, lentils, and chickpeas.

Braise gently for a few min, then add the tomatoes. Add the stock, and bring to a boil. Simmer gently for about 15 min, then remove from the heat.

Puree half the soup, then return it to the pot. Heat and season.

Serve sprinkled with chopped parsley.

Serves 6

Beef, Bacon and Vegetable Soup

This is one of the most delicious soups I have ever tasted, and it's always popular. It's fine to have bacon now and again, as long as it's lean. Don't be put off by the long list of ingredients, as once the initial preparation is over you'll have an enormous pot of heart-warming, vitamin- laden soup to freeze for another day.

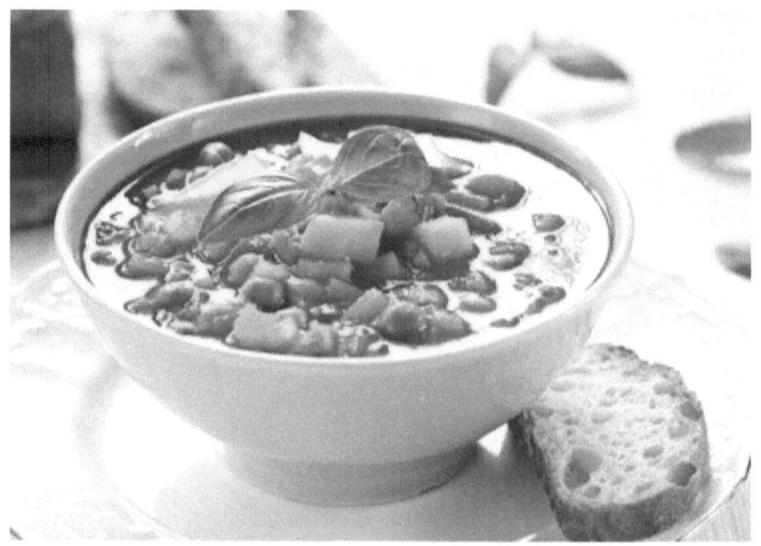

INGREDIENTS:

2 tablespoons olive oil

1/4kg lean bacon, cubed

1/2kg lean stewing beef, cubed

2 onions, chopped

2 teaspoons crushed garlic

2 litres salt-free beef stock

1 can chopped tomatoes

1 teaspoon dried thyme

1 small red chilli, finely chopped

4 medium carrots, peeled and diced

4 medium potatoes, peeled and chopped

2 sweet potatoes, peeled and chopped

1 green pepper, chopped

1 lemon for juice, and salt and pepper for seasoning

INSTRUCTIONS:

Using a big soup pot, heat the olive oil and fry the bacon and beef till browned. Add the onions and garlic and fry until soft. Add stock, tomatoes, thyme, and chilli. Cover and simmer on a gentle heat for 1 ½ hours. Add carrots, potato, butternut, and green pepper. Simmer for another hour or so until all the vegetables are soft. Add a squeeze of lemon juice and season to taste.

Herb and Barley Broth

This lovely soup is made in a slightly unusual way. It's cooked in the oven so that the delicious potato topping can caramelize. Full of good-for-you ingredients such as celery, carrots, and barley, it's bound to become a firm favorite.

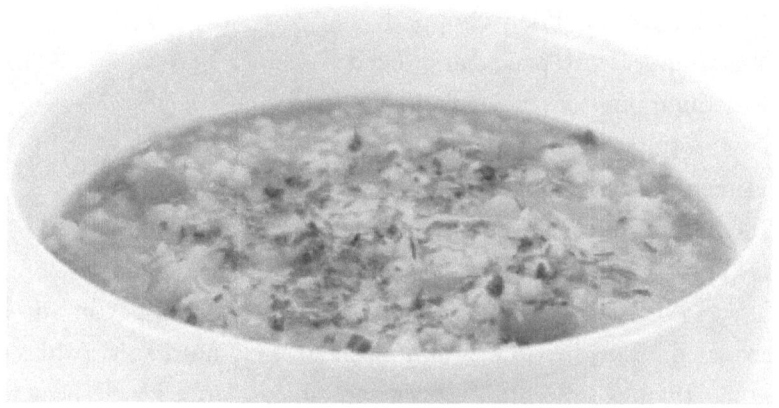

INGREDIENTS:
  100g barley
  3 large carrots, peeled and cut into dice
  3 leeks, cut into short fingers
  3 celery stalks, cut into short fingers
  2 onions, peeled and diced
  4 garlic cloves, peeled and cut into thin slivers
  Olive oil
  Chicken stock, enough to cover, preferably homemade
  2 bay leaves
  1 tablespoon fresh thyme leaves
  6 fresh sage leaves

4 medium sized potatoes, sliced but not peeled
Handful of parsley, finely chopped

INSTRUCTIONS:

Simmer barley in enough water to cover it and a pinch of salt for half an hour. Drain. Set your oven to 180°C. Heat the olive oil in a heavy, ovenproof pot that has a lid. Add the vegetables and garlic and fry until softened. Add the barley and pour the boiling stock over the top.

Put in all the herbs except the parsley. Lay the potatoes over the top of the vegetables, forming a "lid." Don't worry if some of them sink down into the stock. Cover with the pot lid

and place in the oven for 1 ½ hours. Remove the lid. Check that there is still enough liquid.

If not, add more stock. Return pot to oven for another ½ hour to brown the potato top. Remove from the oven. Sprinkle with the parsley and serve hot in bowls with salt and pepper.

Serves 4

Spicy Lentil Soup

This is a warm, spicy soup that is perfect for the winter months. It's also convenient, as it doesn't have to boil away for hours. It'll be ready in about half an hour.

INGREDIENTS:

30ml extra-virgin olive oil

2 onions, peeled and chopped

2 cloves garlic, finely chopped

2 ½ ml ground cinnamon

5ml ground cumin

10ml ground coriander

10ml ground turmeric

500ml red lentils, washed and drained

2 litres low salt chicken stock

30ml tomato paste

1 big potato, peeled and coarsely grated

INSTRUCTIONS:

Using a big soup pot, heat the oil. Fry the onions and garlic until soft. Add all the spices. Add everything else and bring to the boil. Cover and simmer on low heat, stirring now and again. Cook for about half an hour until the lentils are soft and mushy. Puree the soup in a blender. Reheat and serve.

Serves about 8

Cream of Chickpea Soup

This recipe title might sound rather strange, but it makes a light and creamy soup without the addition of actual cream. It makes a quick nourishing supper for those times when you're just too tired to bother with anything more complicated.

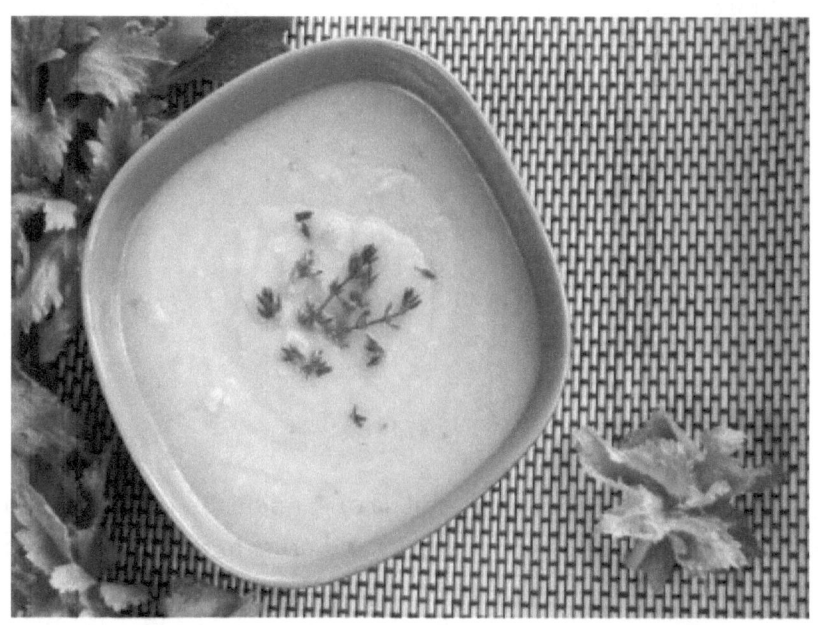

INGREDIENTS:
 1 small onion, chopped
 1 clove garlic, crushed
 2 tablespoons olive oil
 1 can chickpeas (about 400g), drained and rinsed
 1/3 teaspoon dried rosemary
 ¼ teaspoon dried sage
 500ml low salt vegetable stock
 15ml tomato puree

Black pepper and extra-virgin olive oil to serve

INSTRUCTIONS:

Heat the oil, and fry the onion and garlic gently until very soft.

Add the chickpeas, herbs, and 125ml of the stock.

Cook for 5 minutes, then puree in a blender.

Return to the pot, add tomato puree and enough stock to make a creamy consistency. Taste for seasoning and add a little salt if necessary. Heat to boiling point. Serve hot sprinkled with pepper and a drizzle of olive oil.

Serves 4

Meat and Chicken Dishes

One tends to think that meat dishes are a no-go when one is eating for a healthy heart. This is simply not true. Even red meat can be enjoyed, provided you have it in moderation and that it is the correct type.

Focus on using meats as a flavouring for the dish, and not as the main ingredient of a meal. Fill your plate with masses of vegetables, a few wholegrain carbs, and fruit, and then add the meat sparingly as a flavourful treat to finish off the dish.

It's a good idea to choose grass fed organically raised beef, lamb, and pork where you possibly can, and always trim off any excess fat. Focus on using chicken breast rather than the brown meat of the thighs and drumsticks. Where these are used, try to remove the skin, as this is where most of the fat is.

The meat recipes I've provided here include lots of meaty flavour, yet have piles of vegetables, legumes, and other healthy additions. I hope you make them part of your family's menu.

Pork Chop Suey

This well-known American-Chinese dish is made here with lean pork fillet and plenty of vitamin-packed vegetables. "Chop suey" literally means "assorted bits" and in this case they're assorted heart-smart bits! Serve it with brown rice for a healthier version. Yes, pork is acceptable as a heart-healthy option, as long as you use the fillet (tenderloin) which is actually as lean as chicken breast.

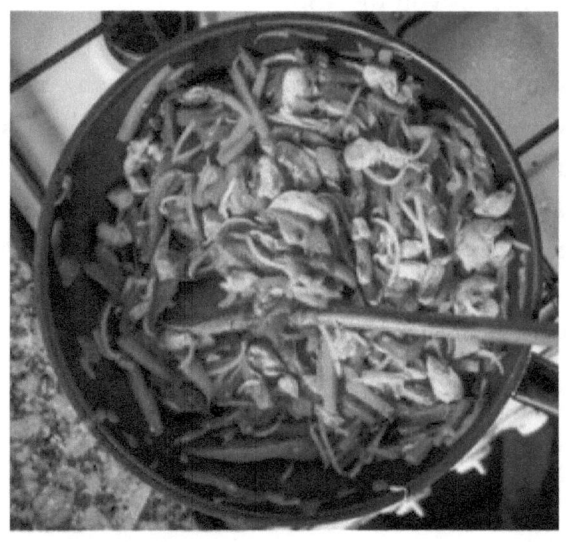

INGREDIENTS:
  4 tablespoons sesame seed oil
  400g pork fillet, cut into strips
  250g button mushrooms, sliced
  1 leek, trimmed, washed, cut at an angle into thin rings
  2 carrots, peeled, and cut into strips
  1 red pepper, seeds removed and cut into strips
  150g soya sprouts
  1 can bamboo shoots (about 450g), drained

75ml low sodium soya sauce
White pepper to season

INSTRUCTIONS:

Using a wok, heat the oil and stir-fry the meat.

Push it to the side of the wok or remove to a dish and add the mushrooms,

leek, carrots, pepper, and soya sprouts. Stir fry all together until cooked but still crisp.

Add the bamboo shoots. Stir the meat back in and add soya sauce and pepper. Serve on brown rice or low fat noodles.

Serves 4

Slow-Baked Lamb Knuckles with Chickpeas

Lamb is a good option if you choose grass-fed lamb. It tends to have
higher amounts of heart-friendly omega 3's than other lamb. Other
good ingredients in this dish are heaps of garlic, some red wine, and
cinnamon. This deliciously saucy dish has plenty of vegetables and
chickpeas too. Spicy and warming for the winter months.

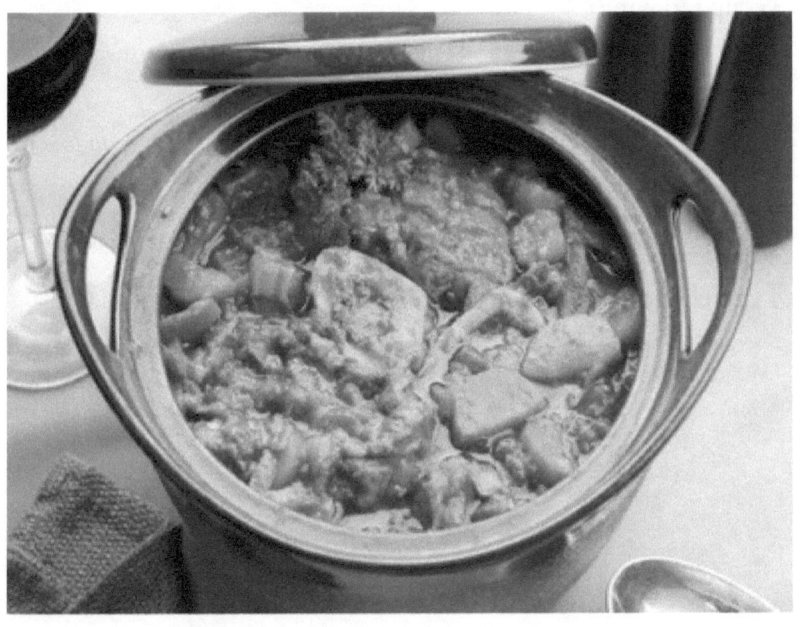

INGREDIENTS:

1kg grass-fed lamb knuckles, sliced
30ml olive oil
2 onions, finely chopped
4 cloves garlic, crushed
10ml ground cumin
10ml ground coriander
30ml whole-wheat flour
1 cup hot low-salt beef or mutton stock
½ cup red wine
1 can chopped tomatoes (410g)
15ml tomato paste
400g butternut squash, peeled and diced
15ml honey
2 cinnamon sticks
4 bay leaves
1 can chickpeas, drained and rinsed to remove salt

INSTRUCTIONS:

Using a big frying pan or wok, brown the lamb pieces in the oil. Place them in a large, deep, ovenproof dish. Add the onions, garlic, cumin and coriander to the wok and fry for a minute, deglazing the pan with a little stock if necessary. Add the flour, stirring to a paste, then slowly stir in

the stock, wine, and tomatoes. When smooth and thickened, add everything else except the chickpeas.

Bring to the boil, then pour over the lamb.

Cover with a lid, or some tinfoil. Bake slowly at 160°C for 1 ¼ hours. Remove the bay leaves and cinnamon sticks. If too dry, add a little more wine or stock. Add the chickpeas, cover again, and bake for 30 minutes more, after which time the lamb should be soft and the sauce thick.

Serve with whole-wheat couscous and a spoonful of low fat Greek yoghurt. Serves 5 or 6

Cottage Pie with Sweet Potato Topping

Sweet potatoes replace the normal white potatoes for the topping here, and olive oil substitutes for butter in the mash. Be sure to use extra-lean, grass-fed beef mince. Then enjoy this lovely shepherd's pie with a clear conscience.

INGREDIENTS:

1 kg sweet potato, peeled, cubed, and boiled till soft
60ml olive oil
25ml honey
About ½ cup fat-free milk
50g celery, chopped (include some leaves)
100g carrots, peeled and chopped
100g onions, peeled and chopped
1 clove garlic, finely chopped
500g lean, grass fed beef mince (ground beef)
2 cups low-salt beef stock
1 tin chopped tomatoes (410g)
Handful Italian parsley, finely chopped

INSTRUCTIONS:

Set oven at 180°C. Mash the cooked sweet potato with 30ml of the olive oil, 10ml of the honey, and the milk. Using a wok or frying pan, fry celery, carrots, onions, and garlic in the remaining oil till slightly caramelised. Add the mince and brown it, breaking up any lumps. Add stock and tomatoes and cook down for about 30 min on low heat till thickened. Add parsley and the other 10ml of honey. Taste and check the seasoning. Place in an ovenproof dish and top with the sweet potato mash. Cover with foil, shiny side in, for about 20 min.

Serves 4-6

Tex-Mex Pasta

Small amounts of cheese are good for your heart, provided that you stay
away from processed cheeses. Cheese contains compounds that can
inhibit the *angiotensin-converting enzyme* (ACE) that controls blood
pressure. The trick is to just sprinkle small amounts of cheese over a
dish, as in this recipe, or to have a small sliver with a chunk of fruit,
rather than eating it in the enormous quantities usually found in the
typical American diet.

INGREDIENTS:

30ml extra-virgin olive oil

1 onion, finely chopped

2 cloves garlic, very finely chopped

1 green pepper, chopped

300g extra-lean grass-fed beef mince (ground beef)

1 fresh red chilli, finely chopped

2 tins chopped tomatoes (410g each)

3 courgettes, coarsely grated

½ cup frozen corn kernels

¼ teaspoon salt

1 teaspoon honey

½ cup grated Cheddar cheese, to sprinkle

300g whole-wheat pasta shapes, for example penne, boiled in lightly salted water

INSTRUCTIONS:

Using a large frying pan, heat the oil and stir-fry the onion, garlic, and green pepper till soft. Add the mince and cook until soft. Add chilli, tomatoes, courgette, corn, salt and honey. Simmer gently, uncovered, till sauce has thickened. Taste for seasoning. Serve mixed with the pasta, and topped with a little cheese. Serves 4

Roast Chicken on a Bed of Mushroom and Pea Rice

A simple weeknight one-dish meal that the whole family will love.

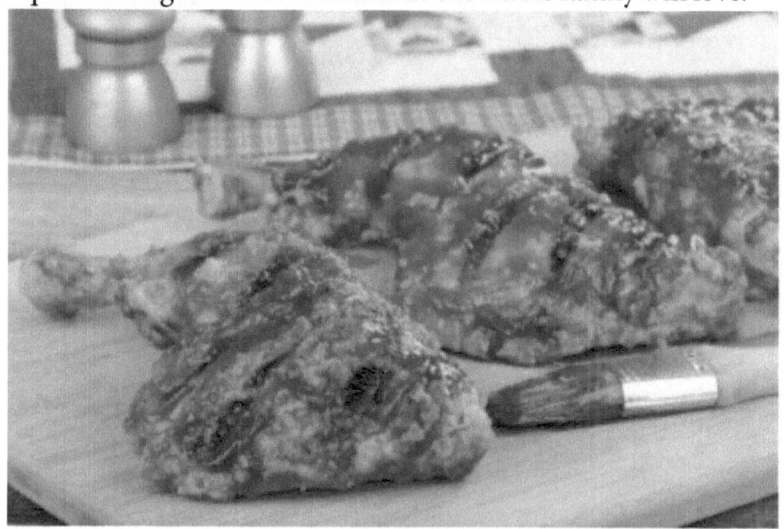

INGREDIENTS:

1 cup brown rice, cooked in chicken stock and drained

1 cup baby peas, lightly cooked

1 young free-range chicken, roasted till golden, then cooled and carved into portions (I use a ready cooked barbeque chicken from the store.)

10ml olive oil

1 onion, chopped

1 clove garlic, finely chopped

1 red bell pepper, chopped

250g button mushrooms, sliced

Salt, pepper, and nutmeg to season

INSTRUCTIONS:

Using a wok or frying pan, heat the oil, and fry the onion, garlic, and red pepper till soft. Add the mushrooms and continue to fry until they are

cooked. Remove from the heat. Stir in the cooked rice and peas. Season well.

Tip into a serving dish and top with portions of the carved chicken. Serve hot or warm.

Serves 4-6

Chicken Strips on a Bed of Roast Butternut and Feta Rice

There are lots of nutritious ingredients combined in this super-tasty dinner dish. The caramelized butternut and sweet red peppers are a winner when mixed with the succulent chicken.

INGREDIENTS:

1 cup brown rice, cooked in chicken stock and drained

4 chicken breast fillets, sliced into strips and dusted with seasoned flour

60ml olive oil

1 onion, chopped

1 clove garlic, very finely chopped

1 red bell pepper, cut into cubes

500g butternut squash, cut into 1cm cubes

30ml honey

Large sprig fresh rosemary, finely chopped

1 round reduced fat feta cheese, crumbled

Handful of toasted pumpkin seeds

INSTRUCTIONS:

Preheat your oven to 180°C. Put half the olive oil with the peppers, butternut and honey into a plastic bag. Toss them around to coat with the oil, then tip them out onto a roasting tray. Sprinkle with the rosemary. Roast until soft and caramelized. Meanwhile, boil the rice in the stock. Drain. In a wok, heat 15ml oil and fry the onion and garlic till softened. Stir in the cooked rice. Mix in the roasted vegetables. Check the seasoning. Tip into a serving dish and wipe the wok clean. Pour in the last of the oil and stir fry the chicken strips until golden and done. Cook for just a few minutes so they don't dry out. Place these on top of the rice mixture. Top with crumbled feta and a sprinkle of pumpkin seeds.

Serves 4

Sweet and Hot Crockpot Chicken

Healthier than the takeaway version, you can make this even better for your heart by serving it with a side of brown rice and some stir-fried vegetables.

INGREDIENTS:

4 boneless chicken breasts, semi-frozen, cut into cubes

1 large red bell pepper

1 bunch spring onions, chopped (including the green part)

1 small can pineapple chunks, drained, but keep the juice

1 garlic clove, crushed

1 small red chilli, finely chopped

1 cup water

2 tablespoons sweet chilli sauce

½ teaspoon salt

3 tablespoons cornflour

INSTRUCTIONS:

Put the chicken pieces, red pepper, spring onion and pineapple into the crock pot. In a jug, mix the garlic, chilli, water, sweet chilli sauce, and salt. Pour this mixture over the ingredients in the crock pot. Cover and cook on high for about 2 ½ hours. In a small jug, mix the cornflour and pineapple juice/ syrup till smooth. Add to the crockpot and stir to blend. Replace the lid and cook on high for another 30 min. The sauce should be thickened. Taste for seasoning. Serve on brown rice.

Serves 4

Parsley and Lemon Chicken Patties on Sweet Potato Mash

This is a light and summery dish to serve with a salad when you want a
light meal that's quick to make. Just remember to make small patties,
and not big, burger sized ones.

INGREDIENTS:

800g chicken mince

1 egg, beaten

¼ cup mayonnaise

¼ cup Italian parsley, finely chopped

Grated zest of 1 lemon

¾ cup fresh brown breadcrumbs

1 onion, finely chopped

30ml olive oil

2 cloves garlic, crushed

Salt and pepper

A small amount of flour and olive oil for dipping and frying purposes

4 sweet potatoes, peeled and chopped

INSTRUCTIONS:

Mix all the ingredients for the patties together in a big bowl with
your hands. Using wet hands, form the mixture into about 8-10 patties,

placing them on a tray as you go. Put some flour into a small plate,
and dip each one in flour, shaking off the excess. Place the tray of patties
in

the fridge to firm up for half an hour, or into the freezer for 10
minutes if you're in a hurry. Meanwhile, boil and mash your sweet
potatoes, adding

a little milk if necessary. Set aside and keep warm. Preheat the oven
to 180°C.

Using a frying pan, heat a small amount of olive oil on high heat, and fry the patties in batches to brown them on the outside. Don't worry to cook them through. Drain them on kitchen paper as you go. Once all done,

place them on an oven tray and finish them off in the oven for 10 minutes. Serve with the sweet potato mash and a salad.

Serves 4

Thai-Style Chilli Chicken Breasts

This makes a lovely fresh, light dinner or lunch dish, which is quick and easy to prepare. It's full of goodness from the lean protein, the colorful vegetables, and the nutty brown rice. I'm sure this is a recipe you'll come

back to again and again!

INGREDIENTS:

6 chicken breast fillets, flattened with a meat mallet or rolling pin

Juice of 1 lemon

Brown flour, salt, pepper

Light olive oil to fry

1 small red bell pepper, cut into julienne strips

1 small yellow bell pepper, also in strips

A handful of fresh green beans, cut in half lengthways

A small bunch of spring onions, cut in strips lengthways

1 teaspoon grated fresh ginger

1 small fresh green chilli, seeds removed and finely chopped

45ml sweet chilli sauce

Cooked brown rice, to serve

INSTRUCTIONS:

Sprinkle the chicken with a little lemon juice. Dust with seasoned flour and fry over high heat in a small amount of oil (about 15ml) until just done.

This will only take a few minutes- don't overcook the breasts or they will be dry. Remove from pan and keep warm. Stir-fry the vegetable strips in

the same pan with the ginger and chilli until cooked but still crisp. Add the sweet chilli sauce.

To serve, cut the chicken into strips and serve on a bed of rice and vegetables.

Serves 4

Pineapple Chilli Chicken Breasts with Stir-Fry Veg

This is another quick, easy, delicious meal that is also so good for the whole family. Use as much or as little chilli sauce as you like, depending on how spicy you like your food. Serve with rice noodles, rather than egg noodles, as one 1/4 cup serving of cooked rice noodles provides a heart

healthy serving that contains no fat or cholesterol, with 195 calories, 45 g carbohydrates and 3 g of protein.

INGREDIENTS:

6 chicken breast fillets, flattened with a meat mallet or rolling pin

60ml low-salt soya sauce

60ml pineapple juice

Juice of 1 lemon

30ml sesame seed oil

About 20ml chilli sauce

2 cloves garlic, crushed

Cooked rice noodles, to serve

Vegetables to stir fry, such as cabbage, peppers, green beans, carrots, onion, and mushrooms, cut into strips

INSTRUCTIONS:

Blend together the soya sauce, pineapple juice, lemon juice, half the oil,

chilli sauce, and garlic in a small bowl. Place the chicken breasts in a flat

glass dish and pour this marinade over them, making sure they arecoated on both sides. Cover with cling film and marinade in the fridge for

half an hour, or even overnight if you like. When ready to serve, heat a large frying pan or wok, add the remaining sesame oil, and fry the

chicken over high heat for a few minutes on each side. Don't overcook or it will be dry. When done, remove to a chopping board and cut into

strips. Wipe out your wok and stir-fry your vegetable strips. Serve the chicken and vegetables on a bed of noodles.

Serves 4

Italian Hunter's Stew

A recipe that would traditionally have been made with a rabbit or hare that the hunter brought home, today this is more commonly prepared

with chicken. Feel free to use hare if you can obtain it though, as it's a lean, heart-friendly meat too.

INGREDIENTS:

125ml brown flour

Salt and black pepper

30ml olive oil

6-8 chicken thighs, skin removed

1 onion, chopped

2 cloves garlic, crushed

1 green bell pepper, chopped

1 can chopped tomatoes (410g)

5ml dried oregano

½ cup white wine

250g portabellini mushrooms, halved

Handful of black olives, stoned

INSTRUCTIONS:

Preheat the oven to 180°C. Put flour and seasoning into a plastic bag with the chicken and toss it about to coat with the flour. Using a wok or l

arge frying pan, heat the oil and brown the chicken on both sides. Remove chicken and place in a casserole dish. Put onion, garlic, and

green pepper into the wok and stir-fry till golden. Add a little wine if it sticks.

Add tomatoes, wine, olives and mushrooms to pan. Season and bring to the boil. Pour this sauce over the chicken. Cover with foil and bake for 1 hour. Remove foil and bake another 15 minutes or so to thicken the sauce. Taste and add a teaspoon of honey if it's too tart, and seasoning if needed. Serve with some cannellini beans or mash, and a salad.

Serves 4-6

Leaner Chicken Pie

This satisfying chicken pie is topped with mash instead of pastry, and the chicken is smothered in a tasty vegetable sauce. This is a dish the whole family will love.

INGREDIENTS:

5 potatoes, peeled and quartered

Low fat milk (about 500ml) and seasoning for the potatoes

200 g spinach leaves, shredded

1 onion, finely chopped

1 large carrot, peeled and finely chopped

125g mushrooms, sliced

Light olive oil to fry

1 clove garlic, crushed

375ml low fat milk

30ml flour, mixed with a small amount of water to a smooth cream

Juice of 1 lemon

5ml hot English mustard

Big handful of parsley, finely chopped

4 chicken breast fillets, semi-frozen, thinly sliced

30ml grated Parmesan cheese

INSTRUCTIONS:

Preheat the oven to 180°C. Boil the potatoes in salted water, drain and mash with the milk and seasoning. It should be quite a soft consistency that will be east to spread over the top of the pie. Add more milk if necessary. Set aside.

At the same time, while the potatoes are cooking, place the spinach in a colander or steamer over the potato pot and steam it till wilted. Cool, then squeeze out excess water. Set aside.

In a frying pan, heat a little olive oil, then slowly fry the onion, carrot, mushrooms and garlic till soft. Add milk and bring to the boil. Thicken this veg sauce with the flour cream mixture, stirring till thickened. Add more milk if it's too thick. Remove from heat. Add mustard, parsley and

some seasoning. Place the sliced chicken and spinach in a baking dish. Sprinkle with the lemon juice, and pour the vegetable sauce over the top.

Top with the mashed potato. Sprinkle with the cheese and bake for about 30-40 min until the top is golden. Serve with a tomato salad.

Serves 4

Tangy Chicken Bake with Tomato and Red Wine Sauce

What a richly satisfying dish this is! It's especially good if served with brown rice and steamed vegetables. It is even better if made the day before and reheated.

INGREDIENTS:

About a dozen baby onions, peeled

15ml olive oil

4-8 free-range chicken thighs, trimmed of extra fat

5ml paprika

1 small onion, finely chopped

1 red bell pepper, seeded and chopped

250g brown mushrooms, sliced

2 ½ ml dried thyme

30ml brown bread flour

250ml low salt chicken stock

100ml red wine

15ml tomato paste

2 ½ ml sugar

5ml Worcestershire sauce

INSTRUCTIONS:

Preheat oven to 160°C.

Place baby onions in a frying pan, half cover with water and a pinch of salt and sugar, and bring to the boil. Simmer for about 6 minutes, drain, and set aside.

Heat olive oil in a frying pan and brown the chicken. Arrange, skin side up, in a baking dish. Sprinkle with paprika. Cover with foil and bake for 30 min. In the meantime, prepare the sauce. Using the same frying pan, add the chopped onion and red pepper, and sauté briefly. Add the mushrooms and thyme and a little stock if it begins to stick. Stir-fry till softened. Sprinkle the flour in, mixing well. Add the stock, wine, tomato paste, sugar, and Worcestershire sauce and stir until the sauce thickens.

Remove the chicken from the oven, discarding any fat in the dish. Cover with the sauce and add the baby onions. Cover again with the foil and bake for another 30-45 min until the chicken is done.

Serves 4-6

VEGETABLE DISHES

We know that we're supposed to eat vegetables and fruit, but why? Well, they're high in vitamins, minerals, and fibre, all of which boost every system of our bodies, from our immune system to our digestive system.

It's recommended that we eat at least five or even more servings a day.

Eat a rainbow coloured variety of them to get the most benefit.

They help with weight control too as it's extremely difficult to overeat on veg as they're so bulky and filling.

A useful guide is to fill at least half your plate with fruit and veg, a quarter with starches such as brown rice or sweet potato, and the other quarter with your protein source such as lean meat or fish.

In this chapter you'll find fresh, colourful ideas with vegetables that will have you coming back for more of these heart loving superfoods.

Fried Rice with Pineapple and Cashews

The cashew nuts featured in this recipe are full of heart-healthy monounsaturated fats. Also the sesame oil and seeds are so good for you.

They contain magnesium, which is known to lower blood pressure, and an antioxidant compound called sesamol, which prevents atherosclerotic

lesions from forming in the blood vessels. You're bound to love the sweet/ sour flavour combination of this quick and easy to prepare dish.

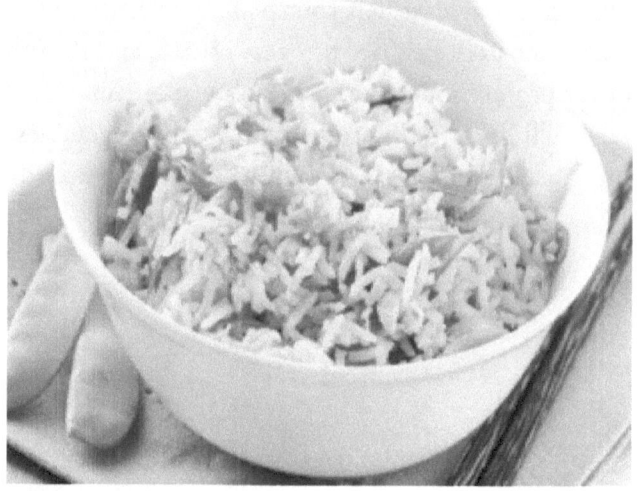

INGREDIENTS:
75ml sesame seed oil
6 small carrots, cut into strips
½ pineapple, peeled and cubed
2 spring onions, chopped
½ cup cashew nuts
250g brown mushrooms, sliced
30ml low sodium soya sauce
30 ml wine vinegar
White pepper to season

1 egg, beaten

2 cups cooked brown basmati rice

Sweet and sour sauce to serve

Spring onion tops or chives, chopped, to serve

Sesame seeds, dry-fried in a pan, to serve

INSTRUCTIONS:

Using a wok, heat 45ml of the oil. Stir-fry the carrots first, then add the pineapple, spring onions, nuts, and mushrooms. Stir-fry for a few minutes. Add the soya sauce, vinegar, and pepper. Stir in. Remove from the wok to a warm dish. Pour egg into wok and stir. Remove when almost set. Heat the rest of the oil in the wok, add rice, and stir till heated up. Replace vegetables and egg. Mix together. Spoon into bowls and garnish with sweet and sour sauce, chives, and sesame seeds.

Serves 4

Potatoes and Greens

Use this lovely vegetable dish as a main meal or as a side, with a piece of salmon to accompany it. Either way, you're sure to love it.

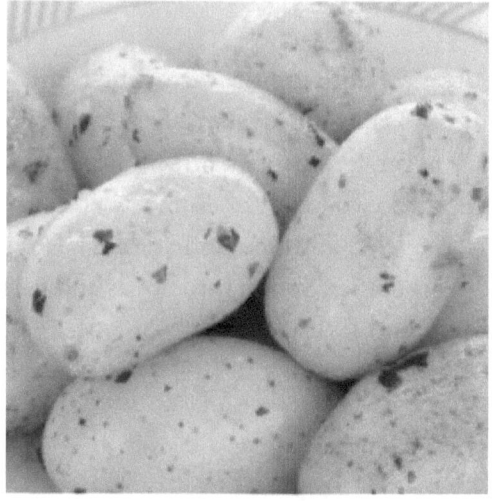

INGREDIENTS:

1kg new baby potatoes

15ml olive oil

400g Savoy cabbage, shredded

250g tenderstem broccoli

250g baby frozen peas

Black pepper

A few mint sprigs, finely shredded

Juice of ½ a lemon

INSTRUCTIONS:

Boil the baby potatoes whole until they're soft. Drain and cut in half once they're a bit cooler. Using a wok, heat the oil and stir-fry the cabbage, broccoli and peas until cooked but still crisp. Mix in the potatoes. Season with the pepper, mint, and lemon juice.

Serve at once.

Serves 4-6

Spinach and Beetroot Salad with Orange Dressing

What a beautiful looking, fresh, salad this is, and it's filled with lots of health enhancing and flavorful ingredients! Serve it on a white platter to show off the gorgeous colors.

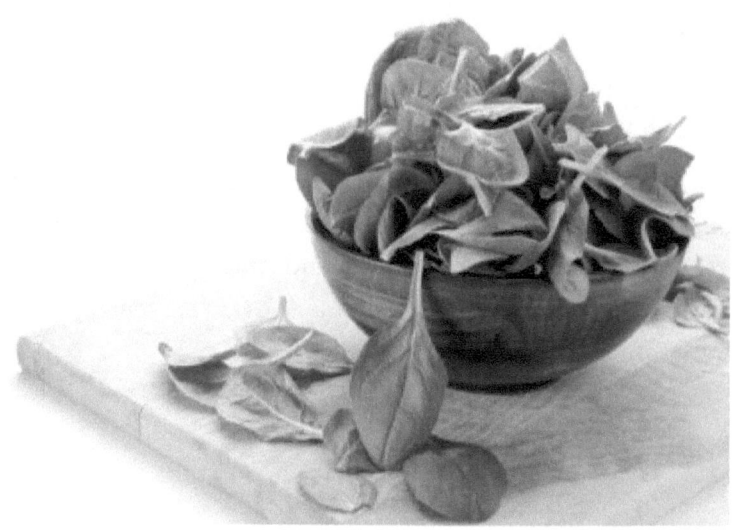

INGREDIENTS:
Small packet of baby spinach leaves, washed and torn into pieces
4 beetroots, roasted, cooled, peeled and cut into wedges
2 oranges or clementines, peeled and segmented
Handful fresh pitted dates, sliced
125g Italian ricotta cheese (low-fat)
CITRUS DRESSING:
Juice of 1 orange or clementine, and the zest of ½ of it
10ml red wine vinegar
½ teaspoon Dijon mustard
25ml olive oil
Salt and pepper

INSTRUCTIONS:

Place the spinach leaves on the platter and arrange the beetroot, orange segments, and dates on top. Using a teaspoon, dollop a heaped spoonful

of ricotta over the top. Mix all the dressing ingredients together and drizzle over the top. Serve at once.

Serves 4

Sticky Roast Sweet Potato Chunks with Orange and Honey

Sticky and slightly sweet, yet so good for you. Could anyone ask for more? This is great with a roast chicken meal.

INGREDIENTS:

1kg sweet potatoes, cut into chunks (leave skin on)

25ml olive oil

Salt and pepper

15ml honey

Juice of 2 oranges (about 100ml)

Zest of the 2 oranges

INSTRUCTIONS:

Set oven to 180°C. Put chunks into a plastic bag, along with the olive oil, salt, and pepper. Shake around in the bag to coat the potatoes well. Tip out onto a roasting dish and place in the oven to roast for about 20 minutes. Meantime, put the honey, orange juice and zest into a small pot and bring to the boil. After 20 min, pour the juice mixture over the sweet potatoes, and return to the oven for a further 10 min or so till soft and caramelized.

Serves 4

Roasted Root Vegetables with Pumpkin Seed Sprinkle

This is such a tasty vegetable dish, with its crunchy topping of pumpkin seeds. It's colorful too, and looks gorgeous on a white platter. All those colors mean it's full to the brim of vitamins, minerals and antioxidants.

Pumpkin seeds are awesome for your health, and contain a variety of nutrients, such as magnesium, manganese, copper, and zinc, all of which benefit those with heart and blood pressure problems. They're also one of the best plant sources of omega 3's. So what are you waiting for? Let's cook!

INGREDIENTS:

400g baby beetroot, washed and boiled till almost soft

350g baby carrots (frozen are fine)

280 g sweet potato, cut into small rounds or chunks, skin on

500g butternut, peeled and diced

200g red onion, peeled

10g thyme, with the leaves picked off the stems

1 garlic clove, finely chopped

Olive oil

Salt and pepper

30g pumpkin seeds

INSTRUCTIONS:

Heat oven to 180°C. Cut beetroot into quarters and place on an oiled oven dish. Put carrots, sweet potato, and butternut into a plastic bag with

the olive oil, garlic, salt and pepper, and thyme leaves. Cut onion into quarters, separate the segments, and add to the bag. Shake all together

to thoroughly coat all the vegetables with the oil and seasonings, then tip out onto the oven dish with the beetroot. Roast for 20-30 min until all the veg are cooked through. Meanwhile, toast pumpkin seeds in a hot dry frying pan and sprinkle them over the vegetables once they are cooked.

Serves 6-8

White Bean and Tomato Salad

We all know that we should eat more legumes, and this summer-fresh Mediterranean salad is a great way to do so. It also gives one a healthy dose of sun-ripe tomatoes and olives. Served with a helping of oily fish, such as salmon or mackerel, it's just what the doctor ordered. You could even turn it into a tuna salad by adding a drained can of tuna chunks.

INGREDIENTS:

2 cans cannellini beans, drained and rinsed (400g each)

2 big, ripe tomatoes, quartered, seeded, then sliced thinly

¼ cup firmly packed fresh oregano leaves

1 small red onion, peeled and finely chopped

2 tablespoons lemon juice

60ml olive oil

½ cup seeded black olives, coarsely chopped

INSTRUCTIONS:

Mix everything together in a large bowl. What could be simpler? This can be made the day before and refrigerated, and is perfect picnic food.

Serves 8

Barley and Sweet Pepper Salad

This is a chewy, substantial salad that works perfectly well as a main course with a green salad as a side, or as a side dish at a barbeque.

INGREDIENTS:

500ml unrefined barley, boiled in lightly salted water till soft

3 garlic cloves, crushed

1 red chilli, very finely chopped

Extra-virgin olive oil

1 big onion, peeled and sliced

5ml ground cumin

5ml ground coriander

5 ml salt reduced vegetable or chicken stock powder

1 each red, yellow and green sweet bell peppers, seeded and cut into strips

250ml baby marrows, diced

30ml white wine

45ml water

60ml seedless raisins or sultanas

Juice of 1 big lemon

Salt and black pepper

INSTRUCTIONS:

Sauté garlic and chilli in a little heated oil for a few minutes. Add onion, and sauté till clear. Stir in spices and stock powder. Add peppers and

baby marrow. Stir fry for a couple of minutes. Add wine, water, raisins, and lemon juice. Cook for a few minutes, making sure not to overcook it-

the vegetables should still be crisp. Check for seasoning. Remove from heat, and stir in the cooked barley. Serve at room temperature.

Serves 8

FISH

It's so important to make fish a regular part of our diets. It's recommended that we have fish at least twice a week. Research has shown clearly that those people who eat fish on a regular basis are less likely to have heart disease.

How we cook the fish is also important for our health, so we want to avoid battering and frying it, or smothering it in rich creamy

dressings, mayonnaise and sauces. Think *fresh* and *tangy*, such as adding lemon and fresh herbs to steamed or baked fish. Actually, the

less we do to fish, the better it tastes, so keep it simple. The top heart healthy fish are what we call "oily fish" such as salmon, mackerel,

tuna, and sardines, but really, most fish are good for you. The health benefits come mainly from omega-3 fatty acids, and other nutrients,

which are a kind of unsaturated fatty acid which help reduce inflammation in the body. Inflammation causes many problems in the

body, not least of which are damage to the blood vessels which leads to heart disease.

I've given you some fresh, easy ways to prepare fish here, which hopefully will make it easier for you to include it twice a week in your diet.

Salmon Cakes with a Yoghurt Caper Sauce

This recipe brings together so many heart-healthy ingredients into one yummy dish. Cannellini beans, salmon, and yoghurt are all so good for one. A light, easy summer meal that you're sure to love.

INGREDIENTS:

2 cans cannellini beans (about 410g each), drained and rinsed to remove excess salt

1 can pink salmon (about 415g), drained

1 egg, beaten

6 spring onions, finely chopped (include some of the green tops)

15ml chopped fresh dill

10ml grated lemon rind

Freshly ground black pepper

1 cup fresh brown breadcrumbs

Olive oil non-stick spray

SAUCE:

150ml plain low fat yoghurt

15ml capers, finely chopped

Juice of ½ lemon. Slice the other half for garnish

2ml salt

INSTRUCTIONS:

Preheat oven to 220°C

Mash the beans. Add the salmon and egg. Mix together well. Add the onions, dill, and lemon rind. Season and mix. Using wet hands to prevent sticking, shape the mixture into patties about 2cm thick. Take the breadcrumbs and press them into both sides to form a crust around each patty. Spray with olive oil spray. Spray an oven tray too. Place the patties on the tray and bake for 30 min, turning halfway through.

Meanwhile, make the caper sauce by mixing the yoghurt, capers, lemon, and salt. Make a French salad to serve too. Serve the fishcakes hot with the salad. Place a tiny bowl of sauce on each plate. Garnish with the lemon slices.

Serves 4-6

Tuna Tart

So simple to make and very tasty, this recipe works just as well served warm or cold. Leftover squares of the tart are great for lunchboxes too.

INGREDIENTS:

4 eggs

60ml mayonnaise

250ml low fat milk

30ml fruit chutney

4 slices brown bread, soaked in water then drained

1 can tuna (170g) drained

1 onion, finely chopped

5ml dried mixed herbs

Pepper to taste

250ml grated low-fat Cheddar cheese

INSTRUCTIONS:

Preheat oven to 180°C.

Spray a rectangular glass ovenproof dish with non-stick spray and set aside. In a big bowl, whisk the eggs, mayonnaise, milk and chutney together. Add the crumbled up bread, tuna, onion, herbs, pepper, and half the cheese. Mix well and pour into the greased dish. Sprinkle with the remaining cheese. Bake for about 30 min until set. Cut into 8 squares and serve warm or cold with a salad. Serve with more chutney on the side.

Serves 6

Fish Bake with Crumb Topping and a Tomato Sauce

A richly satisfying, saucy fish dish, that is so healthy too. Nutritious fish, mushrooms, tomatoes, and almonds combine in a dish you'll want to make again and again.

INGREDIENTS:

FISH:

4 large fish fillets, skinned

Salt and freshly ground black pepper

SAUCE:

30ml light olive oil

2 leeks, thinly sliced and well washed

250g button mushrooms, quartered

1 can chopped tomatoes (about 410g)

Salt, pepper, and a teaspoon of sugar

CRUMB:

3 slices brown or wholegrain bread, crusts removed

1 slice onion

Grated rind of 1 lemon

Handful of unblanched almonds

Handful of parsley leaves

15ml chopped fresh dill or 3ml dried

15ml light olive oil

INSTRUCTIONS:

For the sauce, heat the oil in a saucepan and sauté the leeks till soft. Add the mushrooms, tomatoes, salt, pepper, and sugar. Simmer for about 15

min till slightly thickened. Pour into an oven dish to cover the bottom. Place the fish on top and season with salt and pepper.

Preheat oven to 180°C

For the topping, place all ingredients in a blender or food processor and

blend until crumbly and moist. Spread evenly over the top of the fish. Bake for about 30 min, until fish is cooked through.

Serve with mashed potato and a salad or a green vegetable.

Serves 4

Fabulous Fishcakes

Simple and light, you can use most fresh white fish to make these, for example, hake. These will be a treat for the whole family.

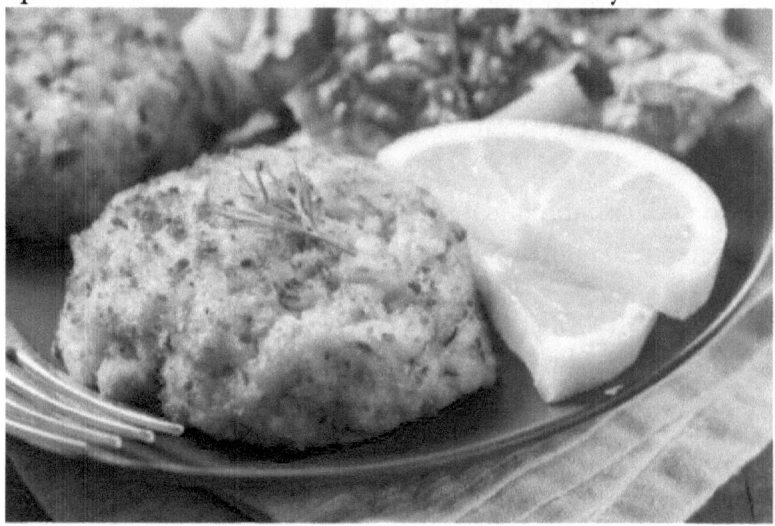

INGREDIENTS:
500 ml fish
2 eggs
dried bread crumbs
5 ml dried mixed herbs
salt and pepper
15 ml finely chopped parsley
1 onion, finely chopped or grated
2 potatoes, boiled and mashed
Lemon wedges to serve

INSTRUCTIONS:

Poach the fish in lightly salted water. Drain and flake with a fork. Beat 1 egg with 15 ml milk.

Combine fish, potato, parsley, onion and dry ingredients.

Shape into patties with wet hands and place on a tray. Chill for about half an hour to firm them up. This is important otherwise they'll break up when you cook them.

Roll in crumbs then in the other beaten egg. Fry in a small amount of hot oil until golden brown on both sides. Drain on kitchen paper towels to remove excess oil. Serve with a salad and the lemon wedges or eat them as they come out of the pan!

Serves 4

Lazy Holidays Tuna Salad

This substantial salad is quick and easy for those days when you really shouldn't be cooking, but is still nutritious and full of good things.

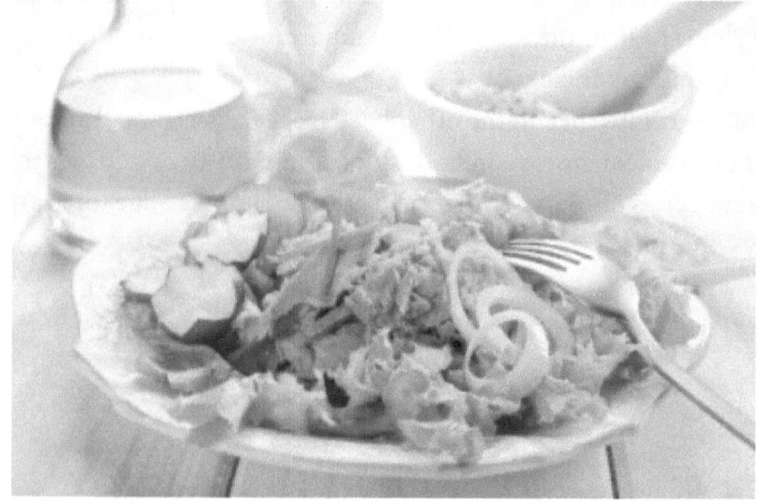

INGREDIENTS:
1 can tuna in oil (about 200g), drained and oil reserved
2 medium carrots, peeled and coarsely grated
1 cup low fat Cheddar cheese, coarsely grated
½ an iceberg lettuce, shredded
1 big tomato, diced
1 small onion, finely chopped
2 pickled gherkins, cut into small dice
DRESSING:

3 tablespoons oil- use the oil from the tuna can and if not enough, add olive oil

2 tablespoons vinegar from the gherkins

1 clove garlic, crushed

½ teaspoon herb salt, or to taste

INSTRUCTIONS:

Using a big bowl, mix the carrot and cheese. Add the tuna, lettuce, tomato, onion, and gherkins. Mix the dressing ingredients and pour over the salad. Done!

Serves 4

SAVOURY TREATS

We all need snacks and treats,besides our regular meals,and snacking can actually be good for us, provided we choose the right snacks! I present you with a few here which are great for in between meals, or for taking to a barbeque or party. They're also ideal for making to add to lunchboxes or for the kids when they come home from school.

Chickpea Dip

Very similar to hummus, but without the tahini, this dip is fresh tasting and perfect to serve on warm pita bread or with whole grain crackers as a snack.

INGREDIENTS:

1 can chickpeas (about 400g), drained and rinsed
Juice of ½ a lemon
2 cloves garlic, crushed
Handful of fresh parsley, finely chopped
2 ½ ml ground cumin
2 ½ ml ground paprika
1 small onion, chopped
Salt and pepper to taste
30ml extra virgin olive oil

INSTRUCTIONS:

Puree everything together in a blender. Taste and season, adding more lemon juice if needed. Serve with wedges of toasted whole-wheat pita bread.

Makes about 360g

Guacamole

A well-known and well-loved dip- creamy guacamole is also so good for you.

INGREDIENTS:

1 small red onion, peeled and finely chopped

1 fresh red chilli, seeded and finely chopped

1 clove garlic, crushed

3 ripe avocados, skin removed and coarsely chopped/mashed

1 ripe tomato, finely chopped

Juice of 2 limes or 1 lemon

Salt and freshly ground black pepper

INSTRUCTIONS:

Mix everything together, and serve with fresh vegetable sticks or wedges of toasted whole-wheat pita bread. Use as a spread on wraps with some shredded chicken breast and lettuce, too.

Spicy Tuna Filling

This is such a versatile little dip recipe. Serve it in a small bowl surrounded by whole grain crackers, or use it as a filling for sandwiches and wraps. You can even use it as a topping for a green salad to make a well-balanced light lunch. Whatever way you choose to use it, it's healthy and delicious.

INGREDIENTS:

1 can tuna in brine, drained

1 small onion, grated

20ml reduced oil salad dressing

2 ½ ml Cajun spice

5ml lemon juice

Freshly ground black pepper

INSTRUCTIONS:

Mix all the ingredients together in a bowl and serve.

Spicy Sweet Potato Oven Chips

On those days when you're just craving a plate of hot potato chips, please don't resort to the greasy, unhealthy takeaway kind. Make these heart-healthy little treats in under an hour in your oven. Remember to use the salt sparingly.

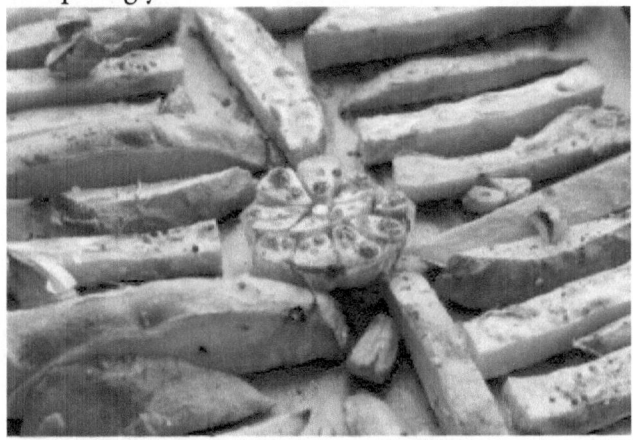

INGREDIENTS:
1kg sweet potatoes
30ml extra-virgin olive oil
5ml cumin seeds
5ml paprika
2ml cayenne pepper
Salt and black pepper to taste
INSTRUCTIONS:
Preheat oven to 200°C. Line an oven dish with baking parchment.

Scrub the sweet potatoes and cut them into chip shapes, leaving the skin on if you wish. Place in a plastic bag with the oil and spices and toss everything together to coat the chips well. Tip out onto the oven dish, in a single layer, and bake for about 45 min till cooked through and golden. Turn them over halfway through the cooking time.

Serves about 4

SWEET TREATS

This little chapter of sweetness includes recipes that are very versatile. What I mean by this is that most of them can be used as snacks, breakfasts, or desserts. We all need a little sweetness in our lives, but just remember that the bulk of it should come from fruits, tiny amounts of maple syrup or honey, and sweet spices such as cinnamon. A little dark chocolate won't hurt either!

Healthier Bran Muffins

Although many people think of bran muffins as being a healthy breakfast option, most are not. They often contain high amounts of refined sugar and flour, and a lot of oil. This version is still satisfyingly sweet, but contains far less sugar and more good things than usual like oats and apples. So go on, indulge now and again. They freeze very well, by the way.

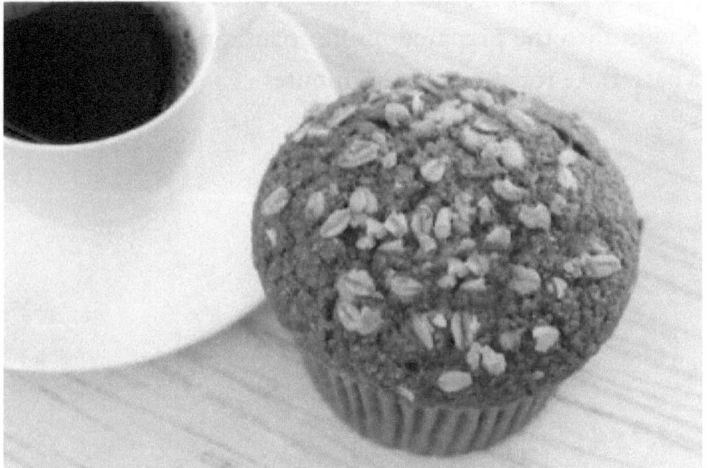

INGREDIENTS:
½ cup light olive oil
2 eggs
5ml vanilla essence
500ml low fat milk
250ml brown sugar
2.5ml salt
250ml whole-wheat flour
250ml cake flour
125ml oats, plus extra for topping
500ml digestive wheat bran
250ml raisins or sultanas, or a mixture

10ml baking soda
10ml baking powder
2 apples, coarsely grated, skin left on
INSTRUCTIONS:
Preheat oven to 180°C. Spray 24 muffin pans with non-stick baking spray.

In one bowl, beat together all the wet ingredients: oil, eggs, vanilla, milk and apple. Mix all the dry ingredients together in another big bowl. Mix everything together. Do not overmix- just mix until everything is together. Spoon into the prepared muffin pans. Sprinkle the tops with some extra oats. Bake for about 15-20 minutes.

Makes 24

Seed Bars

A scrumptious way of getting all those healthy seeds in one bite, while having a treat at the same time.

INGREDIENTS:

250 ml sesame seeds

250 ml sunflower seeds

250 ml linseeds

250 ml chopped nuts (walnuts, pecan, hazelnuts, or cashews or a mixture)

100 g butter

60 ml honey

125 ml brown sugar

INSTRUCTIONS:

Heat nuts and seeds in a large frying pan until lightly toasted.

Meanwhile heat the butter, honey and sugar, stirring until sugar has dissolved. Bring to the boil and heat to the soft ball stage.

Add toasted ingredients and press into a lightly oiled pan.

When nearly cold cut into bars.

Store in an airtight container.

Makes 20.

Sweetened Breakfast Yoghurt

This is a super-simple breakfast dish that packs quite a nutritional punch. Quick and easy for those busy days. Quantities really aren't
important here, and you can make it for just one person if you like. Perfect as a light dessert too.

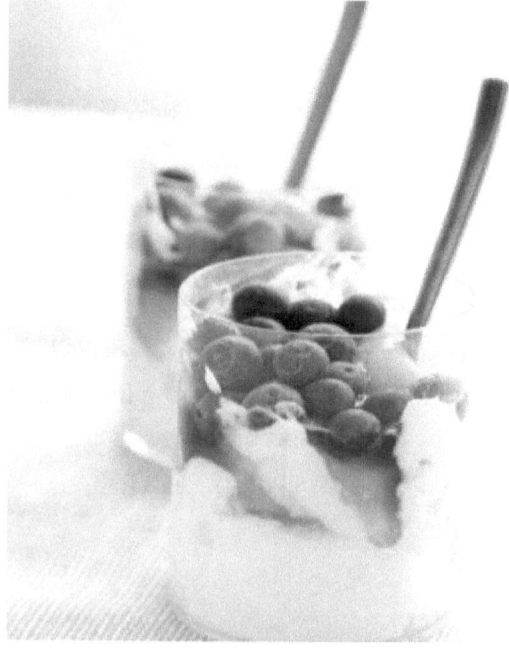

INGREDIENTS:
300g low fat thick Greek yoghurt
1 tablespoon runny honey
2ml vanilla essence
Fresh fruit such as strawberries, mangoes, papaya, berries
1 lime
nuts such as almonds or cashews for the top
INSTRUCTIONS:
Stir the honey and vanilla into the yoghurt, blending together well.
Use about 50g yoghurt for each person. Place it in a small bowl or glass,

top with a generous amount of chopped fruit. Squeeze a few drops of lime juice over and top with some nuts.

Serves 6

Fresh Fruit Fool

Fruit fool was traditionally made with pureed fruit folded into custard or whipped cream. This lighter, fresher, and healthier version has you folding fresh fruit into yoghurt instead. Serve for breakfast or as a dessert.

INGREDIENTS:

3 ripe, soft mangoes, peeled and chopped

1 small pineapple, peeled, cored, and chopped

10ml lemon juice

15ml runny honey

125ml low fat plain Greek yoghurt

A few drops of vanilla essence

INSTRUCTIONS:

Using a food processor or blender, blend together the fruit, lemon juice and honey till smooth. Place in a glass bowl, cover, and chill. When ready to serve, stir vanilla into the yoghurt. Spoon the fruit into individual glass dessert bowls or glasses, place a large dollop of yoghurt on top of each and swirl it through. Don't mix it completely in- you want a marbled effect here.

Serves 4

Better Breakfast Oatmeal

Oatmeal is one of the best things you can add to your diet for your heart and blood pressure. Here it's served with some unusual but yummy toppings, all of which add value in terms of nutrition and flavour.

INGREDIENTS:

1 big cup oatmeal

2 ½ cups water

½ cup low fat milk

Pinch of salt

INSTRUCTIONS:

Place everything together in a pot on high heat, bring to the boil, then turn the heat down and simmer for about 15min until soft and creamy. Stir with a wooden spoon to help the oats break down. If it's too thick for your taste, add a little more boiling water. Serve immediately, as it becomes stodgy if it's left to stand.

Serve with more milk, if you like, and then try these healthy toppings:

Grated 70% dark chocolate and a teaspoonful orange marmalade.

A generous sprinkling of cinnamon (adds a touch of sweetness without the sugar.)

A small handful of chopped almonds and a teaspoon of honey.

Spicy Apple and Cinnamon Squares

A sweet treat to be enjoyed occasionally, this is great for teatime or with a cup of coffee. The kids would appreciate one in their lunchboxes too!

INGREDIENTS:

BASE:

½ cup chopped nuts (walnuts, pecans, or almonds)

½ cup oats

180ml whole-wheat flour

180ml cake flour

125ml white sugar

60ml cold unsalted butter, cut into cubes

1 large egg

30ml olive oil

5ml vanilla essence

TOPPING:

6 cups diced apples, cubed

125ml fresh orange juice

125ml white sugar

60ml cornflour

7ml ground cinnamon

INSTRUCTIONS:

For the base, mix the nuts, oats, whole-wheat flour, cake flour, and sugar in a mixer or food processor. Process till the nuts are finely ground. Add butter and mix in well. Add the egg, oil, and vanilla, and blend until you have a crumbly mixture. Keep 125ml aside for the topping.

Heat oven to 180°C. Spray a baking tray with non-stick spray (about 23x30cmin size.) Press the base mixture into the pan, keeping it smooth.

For the filling, put the apples, orange juice, sugar and cornflour, cinnamon, and vanilla into a big pot. Mix well and bring to the boil. Simmer, stirring, for a few minutes until mixture has thickened. Pour onto the base. Sprinkle the reserved topping mixture over the apples.

Bake for about 30 min, until the top is golden. Cool and chill before cutting into squares.

Makes about 20 squares.

Breakfast AppleBerry Compote

Wow, what a great way to start the day! Prepare the fruit the night before, so that it has time to properly chill in time for breakfast. This makes a delicious dessert or mid-morning snack as well.

INGREDIENTS:

3 apples, peeled and cored

45 ml apple juice

250 ml fresh or frozen blueberries

30 ml honey

2 cups plain low-fat Greek yoghurt, to serve

125ml granola, to serve

INSTRUCTIONS:

Dice the apples and put into a pot with the apple juice. Bring to the boil, then cover and simmer for a few minutes until soft. Add the berries and honey, and cook for another couple of minutes. Cool and chill.

Serve topped with yoghurt and a sprinkle of granola. The fruit will keep well in the fridge, covered, for up to 4 days.

Serves 4

Conclusion

I hope you've enjoyed this collection of recipes, and thank you again for purchasing it.

I know it will be a valuable addition to your recipe collection, and you are encouraged to come back to it again and again, and to make these foods a part of your weekly menu, and part of your healthy lifestyle.

May you be blessed with health and happiness as you make heart-friendly choices!

www.ingramcontent.com/pod-product-compliance
Lightning Source LLC
Chambersburg PA
CBHW022338290526
45785CB00017B/2057